GRADUALLY VEGAN

Lose Weight Naturally

Charles Thornton

I0436538

Legal Disclaimers & Notices

Table of Contents

Gradually Vegan

Before trying this way of life read the entire book before beginning the diet.

Weight Loss

A vegan diet is a plant based; it is the best diet for a long healthy life. The vegan, like the vegetarian doesn't eat animal meat. The difference between the vegan and the vegetarian is that the vegan does not use or buy animal products. Vegans tend to believe that animals should not be used for eating, made into clothes, or rapping around furniture. Starting and maintaining a vegan diet is not difficult at all. People are so use to eating toxic diets and they make many excuses for eating healthy. There aren't many restrictions when eating vegetables, because vegetables are not caloric dense food. A vegan diet almost eliminates the need to count calories.

The purpose of this book is to save lives, save money, keep people out of the hospital, and help people lose weight. *Gradually Vegan* book is geared to slowly change the meat eater's diet to become a vegan. Eating a plant based diet will; reduce many of the diseases and disorders that people die from each year, save money in prescriptions related to the self-inflicted diseases from eating bad foods, and make people lose weight with fast results like they had a gastric bypass.

Week 1

Monday eat you regular diet. Tuesday eat one meal totally vegan and all other meals as you would normally eat. Wednesday eat two meals totally vegan and all other meals as you would normally eat. Thursday eat your regular diet. Friday eat your regular diet. Saturday eat all meals, vegan. Sunday eat your regular diet.

Week 2

Monday eat your regular diet. Tuesday eat all meals, vegan. Wednesday eat your regular diet. Thursday eat your regular diet. Friday eat you regular diet. Saturday eat all meals, vegan. Sunday eat your regular diet.

Week 3

Monday eat all meals, vegan. Tuesday eat your regular diet. Wednesday eat all meals, vegan. Thursday eat your regular diet. Friday eat you regular diet. Saturday eat all meals, vegan. Sunday eat your regular diet.

Week 4

Monday eat all meals, vegan. Tuesday eat your regular diet. Wednesday eat all meals, vegan. Thursday eat your regular diet. Friday eat all meals, vegan Saturday eat all meals, vegan. Sunday eat your regular diet.

Week 5

Monday eat all meals, vegan. Tuesday eat all meals, vegan. Wednesday eat all meals, vegan. Thursday eat your regular diet. Friday eat all meals, vegan Saturday eat all meals, vegan. Sunday eat your regular diet.

Week 6

Monday eat all meals, vegan. Tuesday eat all meals, vegan. Wednesday eat all meals, vegan. Thursday eat all meals, vegan. Friday eat all meals, vegan Saturday eat all meals, vegan. Sunday eat your regular diet.

Week 7

Monday eat all meals, vegan. Tuesday eat all meals, vegan. Wednesday eat all meals, vegan. Thursday eat all meals, vegan. Friday eat all meals, vegan Saturday eat all meals, vegan. Sunday eat all meals, vegan.

By this time you would have seen a lot of weight loss.

Being a vegan requires a paradigm shift away from a meat eater's diet. Many of the western population consume a high cholesterol, high carbohydrates, high fat, and low vegetable diet. This is the diet of the United States and the evidence is the line at fast food restaurants. Being a nurse on a heart failure unit, I have seen the consequences of the United States Diet. What I have witnessed was people coming in for cardiac catheters, bypasses, and heart transplants, because these people had consumed the United States Diet. I believe that eating a plant based diet will reverse many of the symptoms of the United States Diet. A person on hypertensive, cardiac, diabetic, blood thinning medicine should tell their physician of their diet choices and continue to take prescribed medicine as ordered by their physician.

I challenge you to eat a vegan diet to become energetic, thinner, and healthier.

Restrictions and preferences of the diet:

Vegan diet is extremely easy to embrace in almost all situations according to one's preferences, religion, and cultural view that practice against animal violence or other restrictions.

* This diet can be conformed to halal guidelines.

* The diet can be used as Kosher.

* The diet can be modified with low sodium content with the use of more fruits and vegetables.

* Use of gluten free proteins like nuts, beans and lentils are allowed to help those with gluten intolerance or celiac diseases.

Convenience:

The diet is convenient to apply for your weight loss when you have a collection of recipes to make that appeals your taste buds and satisfy your crave for foods you like. It can be done with creativity and effort. The tip is to plan your meal with the use of plant proteins only and not with meat. There are number of recipes available online and also many vegan magazines are available, books are the best source to learn about the diet and trying out of endless recipes to plan your meals and choose from the list of foods. Eating out is possible in this diet if you limit some of the dishes and foods available outside to break your diet. Choose veggie soups, clear broths and raw veggies or fruit salads as appetizers. Steamed and baked veggie dishes for other meals are well. As a dessert, also choose something with natural sweet like honey or brown sugar. Stick to your number of trips and do not eat out unnecessarily. Avoid eating cheese sticks, snacks and heavy appetizers, sweet sugary drinks or creamy dishes. Not all alcohols are approved in vegan diet but only filtered ones are fine, be aware of brands containing gelatin, egg whites, and isinglass, made from fish bladders to avoid and enjoy the rest. This is really a time saving diet in meal planning, calories adjustment, portions, shopping and preparing.

Fullness:

The rule of the diet is to feel satisfied; there is a guarantee to feel full between two meals due to fiber packed grains, veggies and fruits meal.

Taste:

If you prepare or have tried a bland vegan food then do not blame the diet, the trick is to switch to your favorite allowed items when preparing these foods. Add black beans salsa in your wrap rather than steak with fish sauce or mayonnaise, stir fry tofu if you are a fan of frying meat with suitable veggies. Replace meat in cheese meatballs and prepare delicious balls with spaghetti, peas and beans sauce. In the same way, other than salt you can use allowed condiments in your meals for seasoning and easy intake. Smell will be good enough to appeal to you. Few recipes of desserts might be raspberry lavender cupcakes, gingerbread pumpkin seed brittle, cherry-berry peanut butter cobbler, and poppy seed scones to enjoy under vegan limits with best taste.

What is enough for vegans?

Enjoy the guidelines to cope up with a vegan diet without any demise to ensure that a complete nutritious diet is eaten by you daily. Your all risks and nutritional issues will be dealt.

According to Nutrient Reference Values for Australia and New Zealand, the recommended daily intakes of nutrients in which are crucial for vegans are:

High iron and zinc doses

80% more iron than normally required to an individual

50% more zinc than normally required to an individual

Protein requirements equal to meat

Intake of maximum vitamin B12 as required because it is rarely found in foods and also the excess of any nutrient cause issues like deficiencies do.

The reason behind this recommendation is the presence of high levels of phytate and oxalates components present in vegan foods as they disturbs the absorption of the two minerals in our body. The dietary constituents interfere with the absorption of iron and physiological need increase, to improve the digestion and absorption of non-heme iron, consume vitamin C rich foods with iron foods. Any citrus fruits, tomato or their juice can be used to enable iron to work perfectly of storing and transporting oxygen in our body. Use cooking utensils of iron for additional iron and avoid things which work as inhibitors of iron.

Getting Essential Nutrients for a Balanced & Full Of Health Life

Iron:

The vegans must consume iron double than those who are not vegans, for men it must be 32 mg/day and for women 14 mg/day. The sources for vegans are fortified breakfast cereals, breads and soy drinks, firm tofu, legumes, nuts, seeds, dried beans, spinach, chard, blackstrap molasses, bulgur, dried fruits and brown rice. Iron is only easily absorbed from red meat, all leafy green veggies, nuts, raisin bran, prune juice, black beans, sesame seeds, whole wheat bread, beans, lentils, dried fruits and fortified breakfast cereals overcome this issue. Use veggie juices with nuts, fruits and honey if you have difficulty in eating them in other ways.

Zinc:

Like iron, zinc must also be consumed double in vegan diet, 21 mg/day for men and 12 mg/day for women. Good sources are whole-grain breads and cereals, rolled oats, nuts, seeds, legumes, and brown rice and soy products. Phytate in veggies binds zinc also and absorption will not be better, to overcome it if you are not on strict vegan diet, include eggs and meat 2 days in a week. An increase in the recommended doses of nutrients can also be done when there is a growing child, pregnant or lactating women or extremely active individual and requirement of a disease or injury, dietary supplements are used then. When you intended to use meat, use only lean cuts, white meats and skimmed dairy products. They maintain cell structure and integrity of immune system.

Protein:

Apart from common concept, actually vegan diet supplies enough protein. Richest sources are beans, nuts, chickpeas, lentils, soya products, soya mince seeds, nuts and nut butters, peas, pasta, baked veggies, oatmeal, potatoes, corn, cereals, tofu, soya nuts and dairy, rice, maize, pasta, bread and in grains, quinoa and whole grain breads. These proteins are not easily digestible; you need more protein foods in vegan diet to cover the replacement of animal proteins like you get from egg and meats. To mix it with essential amino acids as building blocks for our body and energy, add hemp and soya in your diet plant sources. To rely only on plant proteins, you will get nutritionally adequate diet without saturated fats.

10% of total calories should come from protein–

Normal RDA for protein is 0.8 grams of protein per Kg of body weight

For vegans = 0.10 grams of protein per Kg of body weight

Example:

Based on 1800 kcal diet, 180 kcal from protein

180 kcal x 1 gram/4 kcal = 45 grams of protein per day

Calcium:

For those who are following diet without dairy sources, intake of collard greens, oat puddings, rice, sesame seeds, dried fruits like figs and apricots, spinach, almonds, soybeans and turnip greens should be taken in large amounts. Use calcium fortified soy milk, cereals, orange juice and tofu because oxalates present in veggies interfere with the absorption of calcium. For more options, consult pyramid table of servings given in the section later. We need it for various functions of promoting clotting, teeth, bones and growth. 1200 mg is needed for an individual following this diet program.

Vitamin B2 & B12:

Eggs and meat are active sources of these nutrients, to consume them within plants diet outside weekly dose twice of animal based foods, the vitamin Cyanocobalamin is found as active form in commercial fortified foods only, confirm it and vitamin B2 through nutritional label in fortified breakfast cereals, desserts, yogurts, rice drinks, oat drinks, yeast, meat analogues and soy beverages, do not use inactive forms including tempeh, seaweed and spirulina. They are mainly needed to serve functions of cell division and blood formation. 2.4mcg of each vitamin is recommended per day for an individual. Supplements are advised safely for vegans and those who are striving for weight loss like multivitamin containing these vitamins.

Vitamin D:

This vitamin source is sunlight exposure of 15 minutes daily to hands, face and arms as body synthesize itself but food sources other than fortified dairy products and egg yolks, liver and fatty fish must be used on the days when you are using meat and dairy. Supplements or active form of vitamin D must be used with calcium sources for absorption and prevent deficiency. For winters, use fortified desserts, margarines and skimmed dairy products and supplements when you cannot do this. It maintains normal blood levels of phosphorous and calcium. Take it in the amounts of 600IU daily when you find it hard to complete from other means and are deficient in it.

Fatty acids-Omega 3:

You can get it in rich amounts from fish, plant oils, nuts and seeds. Among the sources best are walnuts, flaxseeds oil, rapeseed oil, soya oils, ground flaxseeds and cod fish oil and liver. Sufficient EPA and DHA is must for human body, supplements must be taken if you are not consuming fish.

Selenium is also needed in traces by our body through meat, fish and nuts, vegan diet provides enough for it but you can add Brazil nuts for it. Use sea veggies and very small amounts of iodized salt to fulfill your iodine needs.

Use grains, veggies, fruits, nuts, seeds, legumes, beans and unsaturated oil foods, the servings for an adult to follow daily are given below, suitable to plan a 1800 calorie diet plan while for children or below 18 years of active individuals increase food servings to double:

Food

Servings/day

Examples sources:

Fruits – 2

1 medium fruit

½ cup juice

Grains – 6

1 Whole wheat bread slice

½ cup cooked grains/beans

½ cup brown rice

Legumes and nuts – 5

½ cooked bean, peas, and lentil

½ cup nuts/tempeh/tofu/meat alternative food

2 tbsp seeds or nut butter

Oils – 2

1 tsp oil

1 tsp soft margarine

1 tsp mayonnaise

Veggies – 4

1 cup raw veggie

½ cup cooked

½ cup juice

Calcium rich foods – 8

¼ cup almonds

½ cup fortified beverage/cereal

1 cup cooked broccoli, bok choy, chard, okra, kale, mustard greens, collards and Chinese cabbage

½ cup soybeans/tofu/nuts

*when using milk and meat products on two days per week, replace 2 servings from veggies and 4 from calcium rich foods to include 1 oz. meat piece, 1 cup milk, ½ cup for other products while 1 whole egg boiled, cooked or poached without salt/sodium rich foods and condiments.

*Add essential amino acids rich foods/supplements 3 times per day, on the days of meat and milk it will be filled with eggs, dairy, tempeh and tofu but rest of the five vegan diet days beans, rice and peanut butter.

USDA recommends these 3 basic recommendations to build vegan diet pyramid for your weight loss:

    Low fat protein sources (limit unsaturated fats)

Vitamins and minerals fortified foods

Eliminate all foods with saturated fats

Meal Planning:

Choose foods with desired sources in variety; mix all kinds of foods equally-veggies, fruits, nuts, seeds, grains, legumes, beans and dairy or meat in traces.

Eliminate refined foods, sodium foods, simple carbohydrates and white sugars.

Only use whole wheat/grain foods with sparingly use of unsaturated oils, skimmed dairy foods, lean meat cuts, white meats and limit foods from commercial sources, packaged, fast foods and prepared or not raw foods.

Prefer low fat foods.

Do not use foods with cholesterol as we do not need it, it is made by our body itself.

Do not use saturated and trans fats for weight loss and diseases. Trans fatty acids in hydrogenated fats like margarines and crackers should be avoided, in a healthy way only 8% of total calories are allowed from these.

Some dishes good for vegan weight loss are:

Macaroni with sugar free fruit sauce

Spaghetti

Veggie pizza

Eggplant parmesan

Vegetable soup

Pancakes

Oatmeal

Vegetable lasagna

Peanut butter & jam

Grilled veggies

Bean tacos & burritos

Baked vegetables

Veggie curries

Vegetable pot pie

Fruit natural drinks

Bread & cereals

Yogurt

Fruit/raw veggie, bean salad

Other foods are:

Millet

Tahini

Falafel

Wheat germ

Sprouts

Tamari

Barley

Carob

Soy burgers

Nut loaf

How to replace an egg in baking and beverages?

1 banana for cakes and pancakes

2 Tbs cornstarch or arrowroot starch

Blend ¼ cup tofu

Ener-G Egg Replacer (or similar product sold in health food stores)

What to use to replace dairy?

Soy milk

Soy margarine

Soy yogurt

Nut milks

Rice milk

Use these foods to replace meat in soups and stews:

Tempeh

Tofu

Wheat Gluten or Seitan

BMI calculation:

To know about your BMI is a first step to indicate if you need weight loss or not. BMI under 19-23 is normal if above 23 then you need a weight loss plan. You should follow a plan for 14 days and then you can take a break for couple of days to continue again and achieve your normal BMI. Here is a quick way to determine your BMI and make sure your weight is normal or you need a weight loss plan:

BMI =
(kg/m²)

weight in kilograms

— — — — — — — — — — — — —

height in meters²

Or

BMI =
(lbs/inches²)

(weight in pounds * 703)

— — — — — — — — — — — — —

height in inches²

If you are not sure about your BMI, consult an expert and take advice about accurate measurements, conversion and exact BMI before following the plans and workout program.

Remember:

Following plans with choice of two dishes, select any one.

Do not fill your stomach, only eat to eliminate hunger feelings and take small portions at a time. Stop eating with a space in your stomach.

Follow recipes completely of veggies and low fat/calories for your good health.

Eat raw veggies and fruits as possible without peeling after gently washing.

Season food as light as you can and use oil as less as you can.

Prepare all legumes properly, wash and pick finely.

Make a food diary and record whatever you eat or drink daily even a glass of water and a sip of juice or a bite of cookie, it matters.

Eat consciously in a relaxing and sitting manner without any stimulation like TV.

Drink daily 2 liters of water, divide glasses of water and drink one after every two hours to take 8 each day. Drink before meals and not after, use slightly warm water with honey or drops of fresh lime, it will burn your fat or reduce your sweet tooth.

To divide the liquid intake:

1 glass as first thing in the morning

1 glass before breakfast

1 glass before mid morning smoothie or snack

1 glass before lunch

1 glass before evening snack

2 glasses before dinner

1 glass between dinner and bed time beverage

6 meals plan is presented here for your ease, do not eat between these and follow timings suitable for you strictly

Use a cup of warm milk to use in bed time beverage when you have your two days of using meat and milk and include in smoothies too

Accompany 30 minutes of strenuous activity daily or one hours of slow activity,

For 30 minutes strenuous physical activity:

Brisk walk

15 minutes of jogging + workout

Yoga/Stretching of each body part 10 times each

Join gym/swimming class

Boxing/any other sport

For one hour of slight physical activity:

Slow walk

Workout

Dance

Light yoga

Basketball/any other sport

Replace meat and dairy twice a week in a manner as stated above.

31 Day Eating Plan

4 weeks-a month's plan is made to help you in losing weight fast and stable without any weakness or deficiency!

Day
Early Morning dose to boost metabolism and fight fats
Breakfast
Mid-Morning Smoothie/Snack
Lunch
Evening Time
Dinner
Bed Time Beverage to ease sleep/digestion (optional)

1
Warm water with juice of a lemon
Fresh Grapefruit or Fresh Apples
Walnuts
Bowl of cooked lady fingers or
Bowl of Moong legume
Fresh Kiwi or Fresh Watermelon
Quinoa and black beans curry with tofu
Plain green tea with cinnamon & honey

2
Warm water with 1 tsp apple cider vinegar
Apple pancake
Strawberry smoothie
Leek, Asparagus & Herb Soup
or
Triple Celery Bisque
Orange and pear
Curried Cashew Burgers
Plain black tea with cardamom & ginger- without any sugar

3
Warm water with juice of a lemon
Fresh Pomegranate or Fresh Plums
Pistachio

Spinach or Sautéed green beans with walnuts
Fresh Oranges or Fresh Berries
Macaroni and veggie lasagna
Plain green tea with cinnamon & honey

4
Warm water with 1 tsp apple cider vinegar
Banana smoothie with nut milk
Carrot, cucumber and tomato sticks
Roasted Red Pepper Subs
Roasted peach
Pasta with Parsley-Walnut Pesto
Plain black tea with cardamom & ginger- without any sugar

5
Warm water with juice of a lemon
Fresh Grapefruit or Fresh Pineapples
Pine nuts
Baked beans with veggies or vegetables and bean salad
Fresh Watermelon or Fresh Kiwi
Orange-Infused Roasted Green Beans & Red Peppers
Plain green tea with cinnamon & honey

6
Warm water with 1 tsp apple cider vinegar
Muffin and a cup of grapefruit juice
Watercress & Pickled Ginger Salad
Baked mix greens curry
Black bean dip with sesame carrots
Pumpkin curry & Romaine Salad (Marouli Salata)
Plain black tea with cardamom & ginger- without any sugar

7
Warm water with juice of a lemon
Fresh Apricots or Fresh Melons
Sunflower seeds or Pine nuts
Poached eggs or Carrot cucumber and beet in a curry
Fresh Apples or Fresh Plums
Roasted Vegetable Pasta & Lemony Carrot Salad with Dill
Plain green tea with cinnamon & honey

8
Warm water with 1 tsp apple cider vinegar
Raspberries and whole wheat toasts
Papaya-Avocado Salad
Beet salad and Pineapple-Coconut Frappe
Almonds
Roasted Vegetable & Feta Sandwiches
Plain black tea with cardamom & ginger- without any sugar

9
Warm water with juice of a lemon
Fresh Plums or Fresh Kiwi
Pumpkin seeds
Stuffed potato with Onion, tomato or veggie stew
Fresh Oranges or Fresh Berries
Hummus and Sundried Tomato Wrap and cup of leftover Curried
Tomato Lentil Soup
Plain green tea with cinnamon & honey

10
Warm water with 1 tsp apple cider vinegar
Green apple oatmeal
Balsamic Zucchini Sandwich and Curried Tomato Lentil Soup
Bruschetta with Roasted Peppers
Ginger fruit smoothie
Red or Green Bell Pepper strips with black bean chili roast
Plain black tea with cardamom & ginger- without any sugar

11
Warm water with juice of a lemon
Fresh Pomegranate or Fresh Berries
Sunflower seeds or Pine nuts
A bowl of boiled spinach with chickpeas
Pears or mango
White Bean Hummus with Fresh Thyme
Plain green tea with cinnamon & honey

12
Warm water with 1 tsp apple cider vinegar

Cereal and mixed berries cup
Oatmeal Banana Bites
Moroccan Bean Stew with Sweet Potatoes
Blue Corn Chip Salad
Kale and avocados salad with Miso Soup with Shiitake Mushrooms
Plain black tea with cardamom & ginger- without any sugar

13
Warm water with juice of a lemon
Fresh Apples or Fresh Papaya
Sunflower seeds or pine nuts
A bowl of black lentils or veggie salad
Banana or strawberries
Tomato curry with garlic rice and veggie cutlets
Plain green tea with cinnamon & honey

14
Warm water with 1 tsp apple cider vinegar
Green smoothie with raw green veggies
Mango salsa
Oven-Baked Tortilla Chips with Orange and Fennel Salad
Gingered melon
Seared Cauliflower with Garlic and Tamari and veggie burgers
Plain black tea with cardamom & ginger- without any sugar

15
Warm water with juice of a lemon
Fresh Grapefruit or Fresh Pomegranate
Walnuts or Pine nuts
Stuffed bell peppers with
Green leaves or Baked potatoes
Fresh Papaya or Fresh Grapefruit
Noodle salad and carrot soup and Collards with Almonds
Plain green tea with cinnamon & honey

16
Warm water with 1 tsp apple cider vinegar
Apricot oatmeal
Fresh spinach and mango chunks
Veggie pizza

Apple and carrot slices
Wrap with boiled beans and baked veggies
Plain black tea with cardamom & ginger- without any sugar

17
Warm water with juice of a lemon
Fresh Melons or Fresh Watermelon
Pumpkin seeds or Sunflower seeds
A bowl of cooked cabbages or beans
Fresh peaches
Corn salad with pasta and noodle cutlets
Plain green tea with cinnamon & honey

18
Warm water with 1 tsp apple cider vinegar
Spinach, Beet, and Orange Salad
Fresh grapes
Stir fry tofu and boiled beans with rice
Oranges and raisins
Mixed pasta and Garlic Hashbrowns with Kale
Plain black tea with cardamom & ginger- without any sugar

19
Warm water with juice of a lemon
Fresh Oranges or Fresh Strawberries
Pumpkin seeds
Cooked mix veggies or mix veggies rice
Fresh apples
Broccoli soup with veggie roll
Plain green tea with cinnamon & honey

20
Warm water with 1 tsp apple cider vinegar
Breakfast burrito
Muffin
Pasta lasagna
Noodle salad
Mixed veggie and bean loaf
Plain black tea with cardamom & ginger- without any sugar

21
Warm water with juice of a lemon
Fresh Apricots or Fresh
Papaya
Sunflower seeds
A bowl of kidney beans with lemon or sprouted cooked legume with
tofu
Fresh Apricots or Fresh Plums
Black Bean Chipotle Burger with Cran-Apple Quinoa
Plain green tea with cinnamon & honey

22
Warm water with 1 tsp apple cider vinegar
Berry blast smoothie and grapes
Lettuce wraps
whole wheat bread or roll, lettuce, tomato, onions, and mustard
Air-popped popcorn
Red Curry Chickpea and Sweet Potato Soup with steamed spinach
(drizzle of lemon on spinach)
Plain black tea with cardamom & ginger- without any sugar

23
Warm water with juice of a lemon
Fresh Kiwi or Fresh Grapefruit
Sunflower seeds or Pumpkin seeds
Whole wheat veggie sandwich
Fresh Pineapples or Fresh Kiwi
Veggie burrito and mushroom broth
Plain green tea with cinnamon & honey

24
Warm water with 1 tsp apple cider vinegar
Cornmeal Porridge
Pumpkin and Tomato Soup with Steamed Eggplant with Garlic over
Brown Rice
Plain black tea with cardamom & ginger- without any sugar

25
Warm water with juice of a lemon
Fresh Oranges or Fresh Strawberries

Pine nuts or pistachio
Broccoli mushroom stew
Fresh papaya
Kidney bean curry
Plain green tea with cinnamon & honey

26
Warm water with 1 tsp apple cider vinegar
Oatmeal with Fig and Mint
Plain black tea with cardamom & ginger- without any sugar

27
Warm water with juice of a lemon
Fresh Apricots or Fresh Kiwi
Pumpkin seeds or Walnuts
Corn broth with veggies and mushroom
Fresh plums
Red lentil or carrot and peas curry
Plain green tea with cinnamon & honey

28
Warm water with 1 tsp apple cider vinegar
Frozen vegan waffles with peaches and maple syrup or cereal with plant milk and fruit
Mango Lime Sorbet or Baked Cardamom Pears
Tempeh dish
Orange slices and whole wheat crackers
Savory French Lentils and almost instant brown rice and side of steamed greens
Plain black tea with cardamom & ginger- without any sugar

29
Warm water with juice of a lemon
Oatmeal with walnuts and raisins
Bean taco
Scallion Pancakes
Spicy Sesame Noodles
Veggie taco
Green veggie curry or green beans curry
Plain green tea with cinnamon & honey

30

Warm water with 1 tsp apple cider vinegar
Green papaya salad and apricots
Veggie sausages
Tuna salad
Crackers
Tofu-Spinach Lasagne
Plain black tea with cardamom & ginger- without any sugar

31

Warm water with juice of a lemon
Veggie casserole
Veggie smoothie
Roasted Vegetable & Feta Sandwiches
Raw fruit salad
Broccoli mushroom stew or Bowl of chickpea curry
Plain green tea with cinnamon & honey

The 31 days will break your ordinary dietary habits and you will shift towards a light life instantly. Combine your meals with whole wheat bread, brown rice or a portion of whole wheat buns or chapatti as you desired.

You need to stay patient in achieving your goal if you are extra over weight and obese. The diet plans are only one part of weight loss and exercise completes it. For weight loss regime, pick according to your preferences and needs. Select easy available options. Assess your measurements and instruct yourself through evaluation every week that how successful you are in practicing and achieving healthy weight loss. Stay motivated, reach to the success by following all the given tips and guidelines. Self discipline is the keep of weight management, only you can do it for your own self. Self-help books are also a great source to know about some dietary tricks and other ways to stay and look fit.

How to prepare legumes?

Sort by removing all stones and pick debris.

Rinse thoroughly under running tap water in a colander.

Soak one cup of flageolet beans and lentils, other beans or chickpea in 4 cups of water for 48 hours, do same with sprouting but change water after 12 hours and rinse again. Do not add any salt or soda to accelerate the process and discard all water before cooking to prevent anti-nutrient factor purines and rinse well.

Soak of coral lentils and split peas are not necessary.

Cook lentils and split peas in a large pot in 4 cups of cold water for 1 cup of legumes, first boil for five minutes and discard foamy impurities on top, they have lectins. Drain water and rinse well then change water and cook for 45 minutes.

Cook beans and chickpea in pressure cooker, after soaking process, add 3 cups of water per beans cup and after steam accumulation in pressure cooker, and cook for 45 minutes. The freshness, texture and kind of beans determine the cooked quality.

Release pressure under cold tap water and open to drain the beans and discard lectins, store them in a glass dish to freeze while cook flageolet beans only 20 minutes.

Once cooked peel chickpea and legumes to make puree in food mill for better digestion, texture and taste because it removes excess fiber.

Tenderness, speed and energy saving are the reason behind using pressure cooker, when using pot, mash them after cooked but use only for beans and not for lentils and peas.

1 cup equals 66g of legumes yielding 15g of proteins=per day requirement of essential amino acid in an adult.

Additional tips:

* Use only organic foods as possible.

* Eat cooked and raw veggies in the ratio of 50/50.

* Choose wisely, daily add one meal from legumes/beans and one from veggies.

* Be sure with variety in each food.

* Do not use canned or frozen foods.

* Use fresh seasonal foods.

* Use salt slightly.

* Use any condiment just for taste and minimum sense appeal.

* Use extra virgin olive oil or cold pressed olive oil as primary oil source.

* Prevent storage of foods, cook only required amount daily.

* Use cooking methods without using oil, grilling, baking, steaming, poaching, roasting, double boiling and boiling.

* If you think that honey is not vegan as an insect product or animal product use raw/brown sugar only to add sweet.

* Diet without physical activity is useless.

* Make a habit of reading food labels.

* Shop only for required foods and no extra packs of chips, jellies and cookies e.tc .

Few handy recipes:

Before working on recipes, know your ingredients to include!

Use these guidelines to choose the recipes:

Totally Avoid:

Meat

Hamburger, steak, lard, etc.

Poultry

Chicken, turkey, etc.

Dairy

Cheese, milk, yogurt, etc.

Eggs

Eggs and products with a high egg content (e.g. mayonnaise)

Following are food categories for you to use for nutritious and healthy meal preparation for your vegan diet weight loss. It will help you to work on basic food replacements with the same nutritional value to use in place of regular foods rich in fats, sugars and excessive calories. You can refer back to the table given below when selecting the recipes for your diet menus.

Fruits

Apple, banana, blackberries, blueberries, cranberries, grapefruit, kiwi, lemon, mangoes, orange, papaya, pear, peach, raspberries, strawberries, watermelon, etc.

Fruits as vegetables

Acorn squash, avocado, bell pepper, butternut squash cucumber, eggplant, green pepper, okra, olives, peppers (all types), pumpkin, tomatillo, tomato, zucchini, etc.

Vegetables

Flowers – broccoli, cauliflower, etc.

Stems and leaves – artichokes, arugula, asparagus, basil, beet greens, Belgian endive, bokchoy, brussels sprouts, cabbage (any type including green, white, red), celery, cilantro, collard greens, green onion, kale, lettuce (all varieties), mustard greens, parsley, rhubarb, salad greens, scallions, seaweed (including kelp powder), spinach, Swiss chard, turnip greens, etc.

Roots – beets, carrots, garlic, ginger, jicama, leeks, onions, potatoes (all varieties), radish, rutabaga, turnips, etc.; also pearl tapioca

Other – corn, water chestnuts

Mushrooms – baby bella, cremini, oyster, Portobello, shiitake, white mushroom, etc.

Fermented vegetables – sauerkraut

Legumes

Adzuki beans, black beans, black-eyed peas, cannellini beans, chickpeas/garbanzo beans, green beans, kidney beans, lentils, lima beans, peanuts, peas, pinto beans, soybeans/edamame, white beans, etc.; also tofu, silken tofu, soy crumbles

Nuts & Seeds

Almonds, cashew, coconut, hazelnut, macadamia, peanut (listed as a legume), pecan, pine nuts, pistachio, walnuts, etc.

Flax seeds, sesame seeds, sunflower seeds

Nut and seed butters – e.g. natural peanut butter, tahini

Nut and seed flours – e.g. almond meal

Whole grains

Amaranth, barley, buckwheat, corn, kamut, millet, oats (raw/old-fashioned), quinoa, rye, brown rice, sorghum, spelt, teff, wheat, etc.

Cracked grains – e.g. bulgur

Flours e.g. oat flour, spelt flour, whole grain flour, whole wheat pastry flour

In breads, pastas etc. – e.g. whole wheat couscous, rice pasta, whole grain pasta, whole wheat pasta, whole grain tortilla or sandwich wrap, whole wheat buns, whole wheat breadcrumbs

Toasted wheat germ, vital wheat gluten, baked tortilla chips, low-fat granola

Herbs & Spices

Basil, cilantro, dill, mint, oregano, parsley, rosemary, sage, tarragon, thyme

Allspice, black pepper, caraway seeds, cayenne pepper, celery seeds, cinnamon, coriander, cumin, curry powder, garam masala, garlic powder, ginger, Italian seasoning, nutmeg, Old Bay seasoning, onion powder, poppy seeds, pumpkin pie spice, paprika, smoked paprika, red pepper flakes

Sweeteners

Wet sweeteners – agave nectar, barley malt syrup, brown rice syrup, fruit syrup, maple syrup, molasses, pureed fruits (applesauce, bananas), preserves and jams

Dry sweeteners – date sugar, evaporated cane juice, raw sugar, Sucanat, stevia, turbinado sugar

Dried fruits such as dates and raisins

Apple juice concentrate, orange juice, other fruit juices

Dairy substitutes

Unsweetened nondairy milk – almond milk, lite coconut milk, rice milk, soy milk, etc.

Plain soy yogurt, Use 1 part ground flaxseed meal to 3 parts water as an egg replacer

Condiments & pantry

Chili sauce, hot sauce, marinara sauce, miso, mustard, dill pickles, non-fat low-sodium salsa, SambalOelek (chili paste), sea salt, low-sodium soy sauce, tamari, tomato sauce, vegetable bouillon/Vegit, vegetable broth, vinegar (e.g. apple cider, balsamic, rice, white)

Nutritional yeast--Baking powder, baking soda, unsweetened applesauce, pumpkin puree, cornmeal, low-fat graham crackers, mint extract, vanilla extract, xanthan gum, yeast

Beverages–drink water

Recipes

1. Apricot pop for breakfast

½ cup walnuts

½ cup dates

½ cup dried apricots

1 tablespoon honey

1 teaspoon cinnamon powder

Orange juice to sprinkle on top

Beat walnuts, dates without pits in an electric beater till a smooth paste is formed. Press this mixture in a small serving dish and chill in refrigerator. Heat a skillet, warm honey and pour orange juice in it, slice apricots and add cinnamon powder. When syrup is formed, remove apricots from it and spread in a plate to cool then spread them over dry refrigerated mixture. Cover tightly and serve when chilled again.

2. Bean Salad for lunch

½ cup soy beans

½ cup scallions and fennel bulb mixed

2 cherry tomatoes

½ inch piece of garlic clove

½ small onion piece slices

1 tablespoon vinegar

1 teaspoon smoked paprika powder

½ teaspoon poppy seeds

2 tablespoon mustard sauce

¼ cup melon chunks

Low sodium salt and pepper to taste

Rinse soy beans and boil to soften. Chop scallions and fennel bulb. Wash and chop tomatoes. Add all these ingredients in a serving bowl with melons. Mix in mustard sauce, poppy seeds, vinegar, onion, smoked paprika and a garlic clove. Sprinkle low sodium salt and pepper to taste.

3. Bean curry for dinner

1 small onion

1 small green bell pepper

¼ cup vegetable broth

1 small garlic clove

1 cup black beans

1 small tomato

1 teaspoon ground cumin

1 teaspoon red chili flakes

1 teaspoon dried oregano

2 tablespoon cilantro

¼ cup tomato paste

Pepper to taste

½ cup tofu

Chop onion and tomato, cut bell pepper into dices and mince garlic clove. Heat a tablespoon of broth in a pan and fry onions and tomatoes in it with garlic clove. Mix all spices and herbs then fold tofu and pour tomato paste. Let the dish simmer for two minutes. In the meanwhile, boil beans in a pan and drain. Toss boiled beans in pan mixture and it is prepared to serve in a serving bowl with a scallop of plain soy yogurt.

4. Pasta mix bowl

¼ cup raw whole wheat pasta

¼ cup minced rhubarb

1 tablespoon low sodium soy sauce

1 teaspoon honey

1 tablespoon garlic paste

1 tablespoon grated fresh ginger

1 teaspoon pepper

Bring water in a pan to boil and boil pasta, when done, drain and spread in a plate to cool. Take a serving bowl and mix rhubarb with honey, garlic, ginger, soy sauce and pepper. Toss pasta in ingredients mix in bowl and eat fresh.

5. Oats and veggie mix dish

½ cup rolled oats

½ cup turnip chopped and peeled

¼ cup drained lentils

¼ cup raisins

½ of a small onion

1 tablespoon red pepper flakes

1 teaspoon black pepper

½ teaspoon white pepper

1 clove of garlic

1 tablespoon old bay seasoning

1 tablespoon nonfat-low sodium salsa

¼ cup quinoa

Mince oats and garlic clove finely, slice onion and raisins. Boil quinoa and lentils with oats at a high flame. When a smooth mixture is formed, remove all liquid and pour all mixture in a serving bowl. Boil turnip till soften. After the mixture is cool, mix all spices and seasonings. Add onions, raisins, garlic and cooked turnip. Serve together for breakfast.

6. Whole wheat wrap

½ cup tofu

¼ cup mushrooms

1 red bell pepper

A handful of chopped green pickled olives

2 slices of whole grain bread/whole wheat tortillas

1 tablespoon of olive oil

1 teaspoon cayenne pepper

¼ cup kiwi

A handful of pine nuts

1 teaspoon basil

A tablespoon of cooked buckwheat

4 tablespoons of vegetable bouillon

2 tablespoon tomato sauce

Stir fry tofu in olive oil. Chop mushrooms and bell pepper. Chop kiwi, nuts and mix all together in a bowl with pepper, basil and sauces. Toss in the olives. Take bread slices and insert in the center, spoons full of prepared mixture, then make a roll to eat.

7. Fruit salad

1 small papaya

1 teaspoon ginger powder

1 tablespoon lime

A pinch nutmeg

A pinch sage

Pinch tarragon

½ teaspoon poppy seeds

¼ cup baked tortilla chips

¼ cup grapefruit pulp

Few pecans

Few boiled white beans

Few Swiss chard

Cut papaya in bite size chunks, chop Swiss chard, tortilla chips, pecans and toss into beans and grapefruit pulp. When mixed finely, take a serving bowl and combine all ingredients then sprinkle poppy seeds, garlic powder, herbs and lime to give a taste. Provide this recipe to guests also.

8. Mixed veggies

1 small potato

A handful of peas

½ piece of carrot

½ small size onion slices

½ piece of capsicum

A sprout of green onion

2 tablespoon olive oil

1 teaspoon black pepper

1 teaspoon ginger paste

1 teaspoon garlic paste

1 teaspoon cumin powder

1 teaspoon low sodium salt

1 teaspoon oregano

Prepare all vegetables, wash and peel them, chop potato, capsicum, onion and carrot. Boil peas, potato and carrot one by one. Chop green onion and heat in a pan. Sauté all prepared vegetables and add ginger and garlic paste with all seasonings. Serve with fresh chopped coriander and mint garnish.

9. Eggplant Curry

2 eggplants

2 teaspoon onion paste

1 teaspoon black pepper

½ teaspoon low sodium salt

2 tablespoon tamari tomato sauce

2 tablespoon sesame oil

Wash and peel eggplants. Cut eggplants in very small pieces and grate them thick. Heat oil in a pan and fry onion paste and tamari tomato sauce for five minutes on a low flame, and then add eggplants. When they become soft and brown, mix seasonings and leave with cover for 5 minutes, add water to save the dish from getting burnt. Serve when soft and dry form is available.

10. Fruit bowl

1 teaspoon fresh oregano

½ cup green grapes without seeds

A pinch of sea salt

1 tablespoon olive oil

2 tablespoon minced chives

¼ cup cooked lentils

¼ cup orange juice

A handful of mixed nuts

¼ avocado chunks

Prepare lentils of your choice, boil and drain. If grapes are big in size, cut them in halves. Chop nuts and chives. Take a serving bowl, put avocado, grapes, chives, lentils and combine them well with oregano, nuts, orange juice, salt and olive oil to serve.

11. Bean soup

¼ cup dried baby lima beans

3 cups of water

1 teaspoon natural peanut butter

1 teaspoon sea salt

1 teaspoon lime juice

1 chipotles in adobo sauce

½ onions

½ clove garlic

Slice onion and garlic. Boil beans for 20 minutes in water. When soft, leave to simmer for 15 minutes. In the meantime, add chopped onions and garlic. Squeeze lime juice, add salt and mix in the butter with chipotles in cooking pot of beans. Serve after few minutes when thick.

12. Veggie Lasagna

1 garlic clove

A pinch of dried oregano

A pinch of dried basil

1 teaspoon sea salt

1 teaspoon red chili flakes

1 teaspoon crushed black pepper

¼ cup dill pickle

¼ cup mushrooms

1 teaspoon olive oil

½ cup lasagna noodles

¼ cup marinara sauce

¼ cup fresh baby spinach

¼ cups mixed bell peppers

1 small onion

1 cup plain soy yogurt

Chop garlic clove, bell peppers, mushrooms and onion. Boil noodles with oil for five minutes and drain. Boil baby spinach and layer them in a flat glass platter with sides, drizzle marinara sauce over them and spread oregano, basil, salt, pepper, chili flakes with mushrooms, pickle and onions. Spread yogurt at the top and serve.

13. Veggie burger

1 tablespoon white vinegar

1 whole wheat bun

1 small eggplant

1 tablespoon olive oil

Sea salt and ground black pepper to taste

1 tablespoon lemon juice

1 teaspoon ground cumin

1 small garlic clove

1 small lettuce leaf

1 small tomato

½ of the small cucumber

Grill bun over skillet with brush of oil. Wash and peel eggplant, cut in small chunks and then boil. Chop garlic clove and lettuce leaf. Wash and chop tomato, peel and cut cucumber in small cubes. In a small bowl mix boiled eggplant with lemon juice and vinegar and seasonings. Over the warm bun, place seasoned eggplant and vegetables. Cover and eat fresh.

14. Lunch crunch

¼ cup roasted peanuts

2 tablespoon hot sauce

1 teaspoon paprika

¼ cup cauliflower

¼ cup cabbage

2 tablespoon rice vinegar

½ cup mixed fruit chunks

Chop peanuts and boil cauliflower. Heat cabbage over skillet but be careful to maintain the crunch. Chop all fruits chunks you took. Possibly consider 3-4 sweet fruits. Mix vinegar, hot sauce and paprika in a serving bowl. Toss peanuts, boiled cauliflower, cabbage and fruits one by one in mixture of bowl and serve.

15. Greens under chapatti

2 cup of boiled mixed green veggies

1 cup millet flour

A pinch of carom seeds

4 tablespoon olive oil

1 tablespoon red chili powders

Low sodium salt to taste

Mix all ingredients in bowl except oil and flour to make a filling for chapattis. Knead flour with water in dough and create 2 round chapattis of same size, fill prepared batter in center and close as one. Heat a flat pan and cook over medium fire, turn sides, apply oil and serve hot when golden brown.

16. Peel green

This smoothie is a mix of fruits and vegetables for a refreshing but filling smoothie in green hue with richness in Vitamins A, C, K, B2 and B3. It accelerates the absorption of calcium in your body and makes you feel full for several hours. This drink is also a source of providing you minerals including copper, magnesium, manganese, phosphorus, potassium and zinc, Omega-3s, protein and antioxidants. You might substitute green veggies and fruits in this recipe of your choice to create a tasty green smoothie. This recipe will make 2 medium glasses but quantity can be managed for different amount of servings. This smoothie also contains 122% RDA of iron.

2/3 cup pulp of mango

1 small banana

1 whole cucumber sliced

A head of green lettuce leaf

1 cup chopped dandelion greens

A teaspoon of ground flax seeds

1 glass of water

17. Swiss green meal replacement

This recipe is full of fiber and have ample amount of protein and high in anti-oxidants. This smoothie is good in increasing immune system and proves excellent to use as meal replacement. Around 18 grams of protein and 22 grams of fiber are present in total beverage which makes two servings. 25% of calcium RDA and 5 grams of iron is also present in it. It has calories up to 200 only. It is not only a simple recipe to produce beverage and a liquid base of the green smoothie serves as an easy to drink medium and saves your chewing activity. The flavors of fruit and power of vegetables serves as a great mixture.

1 cup kale

1 ½ cups of water

1 cup baby spinaches

½ cup kiwi fruit

2 plums

½ cup orange pulp

18. Nutritional smoothie

This smoothie is slightly heave and balanced in taste, citric fruits and juice makes this smoothie balanced with bland green but fresh vegetables. It contains only 212 calories with 12 grams of protein. A dose of vitamin A, calcium, phosphorous and potassium is contributed in it by fruits. Manganese traces are also given by this smoothie who is perfect for your connective tissues and building of bones. Spinach is bland but awesome enough to add on fiber and rich nutrients in your meal replacement green smoothie. This smoothie is a good source of rich nutrients to stay in your body for long term. Vitamin C as an antioxidant will be proved fine to deal with your food taste and need.

½ cup pineapple chunks

1 cup apple juice (add with derived roughage)

¼ cup mint leaves

¼ cup spinach

A drop of vanilla extract

2 tablespoons of plain soy yogurt

Ice cubes to chill

½ cup water

19. Protein smoothie

This is a protein smoothie; it is extremely high in energy and less in calories. It has 32.1 grams of protein in it. Combination of fruits in this smoothie is perfect for the flavor and to use as a meal replacement drink. It makes only one glass and prepared in only five minutes. Calories are present in fewer amounts and have fiber of around 5.1 grams. This is equally good to use after workouts and is yummy to drink. It is also good in sodium content. Blend the smoothie until smoothen and avoid the use of food products which are not healthy. Many variations are possible in this recipe it will stay delicious. Proteins served as building blocks of human body. It is good for the functioning of immunity systems. They are helpful in increasing the lean body mass which is utilized in tearing of tissues during exercise whether doing for weight loss or healthy lifestyle.

½ cup plain low fat yogurt

½ cup peach chunks

½ cup plain soymilk

1 tablespoon protein powder

½ cup kiwi fruit

20. Hot mix vegetables with tomato paste

2 large potatoes

1 large carrot

¼ cup of peas

1 teaspoon salt

2 teaspoon paprika powder

½ teaspoon turmeric powder

1 teaspoon cumin seeds

1 pinch red chili flakes

1 teaspoon garlic paste

1 teaspoon ginger paste

1 small onion

½ cup cooked tomato paste

1 tablespoon olive oil

Wash and peel potatoes and carrots. Boil potatoes, carrots and peas till half cooked. Peel onions and cut into cubes. Hot oil in a cooking pan and sauté onions, when colorless add ginger and garlic paste, salt, cumin seeds, chili flakes, paprika and turmeric powder. Stir well. Add some water about quarter cup of water to mix the spices and fold cooked vegetables in the pan. Cook till the water dries and serve with bun after topping the dish with tomato sauce evenly. Keep the consistency smooth, nor thick neither thin.

21. Berry Smoothie

½ cup mixed berries

¼ cup chard

1 cup water

1 dragon fruit

¼ cup romaine lettuce

1 nectarine

22. Green smoothie

1 ripe persimmon

1 cup celery

1 small ginger piece

¼ cup grapes

1 cup water

Ice as needed

23. Sunset smoothie

¼ bunch of fresh basil

1 cup kale

¼ cup sundried tomatoes

1 garlic clove

¼ cup fresh dill

1 cup water

Ice as required

24. Fruit and veggie superstar

A pinch of turmeric powder

1 tsp lemon juice

1 cup chilled water

1 cup apple chunks

1 stalk of celery

¼ cup parsley

25. Smoothie with seed energy

¼ cup soy milk

¼ cup vanilla almond

1 tsp flax seeds

1 tsp natural flaked coconut

1/3 cup water

¼ cup baby spinach

26. Triple L smoothie

½ cup parsley

1 tbsp. lemon juice

1 cup milk

1 cucumber

¼ cup melon

27. Legume puree

Cups of cooked chickpea 2

Cups of green veggie, squash or leeks

Spices and Flower Sea salt to season

Blend the ingredients and then heat in oven at 300F for 25 minutes and it is ready but if you need to make soup then mix veggie broth in the puree after preparation with right consistency.

28. Pumpkin seed spread

Mix 2 tablespoons of ground pumpkin seeds with flower sea salt and spices. Combine 1 ripe avocado or well cooked broccoli florets with tomato purée and apple butter and stir with a fork.

29. Hummus to use as sauce in wraps/burritos

Mix spices, herbs and mustard tsp with a tsp of lemon juice and add with onion powder in a cup of cooked lentils to for a smooth paste, add water in a mixture for desired paste consistency.

You can store it in freezer for only 7 days.

30. Hulled Barley

Rinse and soak 1 cup of hulled barley for 24 hours. Drain and mix with 3 cups of cold water in a pressure cooker. Cook on medium heat for 30 minutes after steam accumulated in the pressure. Release pressure and place under cold tap water. Drain the hulled barley after opening the cooker and store in an air tight jar to use under 4 days only.

31. Buckwheat

Simmer 12oz water. Rinse a cup of white buckwheat and add to hot water, boil and cover to reduce the heat to minimum. Cook 15 minutes. Remove lid and cook until all of the water has evaporated. Do not use pressure cooker.

32. Wild rice

Rinse one cup of the rice in water and add a cup of water in pressure cooker to cook rice, when boil then close lid and steam for 35 minutes at medium heat. Remove and drain to serve.

33. Quinoa

If as usual the bitter grain covering is washed prior to buying then rinse well and dry till water becomes clear. Simmer 2 cups of water for a cup of quinoa and simmer 15 minutes till they tender. Use toasting for a nutty taste in a hot dry pan before cooking and after rinsing.

34. Mustard

Blend 2 oz. of mustard seeds (Canadian) with ¼ tsp of flower sea salt and mix lemon juice about 3 oz. and process till creamy. Store in a jar in a refrigerator, this will become thick after 24 hours.

Fitness Programs

Following a fitness program and adoption of a fitness plan is always good in attaining healthy weight and losing weight without any issue. It is good for a healthy lifestyle and overall health.

Something to consider before start!

Evaluate your fitness level to record that how fit you are, what is your score and measurements against required measures for your progress analysis. For aerobic fitness, muscular flexibility and body composition record:

Pulse rate at 1 mile walk before and after

How many pushups can be done by you at a time?

How far can you move forward with legs straight on floor in front of you?

Circumferences of your waist, abdomen and hip bone

Your Weight and height

Design or select your plan:

Whether you work out daily and does exercise whole day but still you need a plan made to assist you and represent your fitness plan, here are the points to keep in mind-

What are your goals? Do not start a program without any goal that what you actually wants to achieve, which body parts you need to tone more and how much weight to reach you are looking for. Hit the targets with your goals. What is your inspiration for doing this exercise? Marathon or champions, Clear goals will gauge your process well.

For the creation of a balanced routine, normally the aim of moderate-intensity aerobic activity is to do totally 150 minutes or you can do 75 minutes of vigorous aerobic activity, it can be divided daily for a whole week or few days a week for training as strength.

If you are a newbie, go on a plan at your own pace. When just beginning, progress slowly and cautiously especially in a specific medical condition simply consult your physical therapist. And take design which gradually improves your range of motion and endurance.

Choose daily activity plan or break as daily routine based on the amounts of your pushups. Build your exercise plan as a challenge, schedule easy workouts and timings. Set reminders to let you know when to walk and start physical activity, do not schedule any other activity at that time. Leave your social busy meetings and TV shows; try not to eat immediately after exercise or before doing it.

Include various activities in your plan or follow a plan in which you get exercises from all perspectives, the categories of activities and target areas are all concerned to improve you in some way or the other. If you have extra fat on thighs then increase number of pushups to that part or if you do slight yoga then your mind will relax and if you include dance steps you will enjoy. Switch to music and spice up your boring work for better results. If you feel this training is not good for you then you will not get enough benefits and end up in a failure, might be gain in weight or something worst.

Do not take it easy and allow time for yourself to recovery, when you start intensely, you will not get it for long and muscles become sore or joints will be injured. Take rest between sessions and rest for fast recovery. Cross training will remove your boredom and keep you fresh, try variety of activities to prevent damage otherwise you might start with pulling your thigh too much and next day you will be unable to do exercise for next couple of days too.

Put everything you try in a diary and stay on track, it will encourage you as a written plan always work for you. Assemble your equipment; buy athletic shoes, dumbbells, ropes, and a ball, punching pad, inflatable mattress, staircase and whatever you need according to what you have in your plan.

Listen to your body and try to be as flexible as your muscles allow you, be creative but try everything slowly. Monitor your progress and when your stamina improves, you will feel a change in your power and activity level. Break things into parts and stay as easy as you can to run and stay determined at your plan.

More than one type of exercises are given here in the sample plan for each body part to stress on, choose any one from and adopt to try in a day as many times each as you can.

Face

Here are some of the yoga exercises for face, they are easy and makes your face slim.

Orbicularis oris muscle- as the name suggested, this works on the face muscles around the mouth and both sides of the cheeks. Close your mouth and press lips together, blow air under one cheek and count till ten with holding the air, after ten counts transfer the air to the other cheek and then transfer from right cheek to left and continue till the number of times you can preferably 10 times or 15. It is highly effective to remove the chubbiness of the cheeks.

This is also a simple exercise for facial muscles toning; inhale air with your mouth and transfer air from one cheek to another like you are doing mouth washing and continue few times. Make O shape with your mouth and exhale air out after each time of doing this exercise.

This is called slimming fish face, you need to suck your lips and cheeks together and then try to do smiling. Hold this face position for almost 10 seconds and repeat at least 5 times.

It is simple enough, hold your mouth open as much as you can and you will feel stretch, continue doing it. All facial muscles will be toned.

Here is the sunken cheeks exercise for face, suck your cheeks and hold for 15 seconds, then release, continue and repeat. If this position is hard for you, you can use any straw to suck on without any liquid to drink, just pretend like drinking with full face power. This reduces cheek fat and with regular practice, you will get a sculptured face.

Smile as wide as you can to tighten your face muscles, hold this position for few seconds and relax. Repeat 20 times a day.

These exercises also make you younger and beautiful with glowing and brighter skin. There will be no wrinkles appear earlier on your skin.

For eyes, boost the skin around eyes through placing your index fingers on both eyes at the outer corner and pulls it gently upwards like cheeks pull up during smile and your eyes skin will be firm and lines removed.

Chin

Firm skin will determine your jaw line and you will smile and appear more confidently. These exercises remove excess fat and double chin. This appears often in weight gain but sometimes face is only big in size as compared to other body parts. The appearance will be improved, include the following lifts.

The chin lift exercise stretches the neck and throat too. Perform it in standing or sitting position. Start tilting your head back till you look clearly at the ceiling and do like you is kissing the ceiling and holds the position for five seconds. Repeat it 5-10 times.

Your jaw lines and cheeks will be tones in this way. Look to the ceiling by lifting face up as up as you can that your face muscles will pull and blow out air from your mouth.

Another one is to pull as much air as you can in your mouth and your mouth starts to sink the cheeks and then gradually release air to tighten your face and jaws.

Your face will be leaner too with chin, try moving of lower lip over upper as much as you can even close to the nose and hold on for few seconds then repeat. The strain on your jaw will tone your jaw line and double chin very well. Engage your face muscles in a row about 5 times and hold your lips together.

Neck roll is another way to release tension on shoulders and ease neck pain with double chin loss. Stand or sit with your spine erect and inhale gently by turning your head at one side and till chin and shoulder look in a same line and then slowly exhale while your face will be straight again to the front. Perform same on the other side of the face and continue 10 times daily.

In jaw release, sit or stand with erect spine and inhale deeply from nose and exhale slowly from nose with lips tightly closed together, move jaws as you are chewing. After exhaling, relax the tongue at the back of lower teeth. Repeat 5-10 times.

Neck

Neck and jaws exercises are almost same because these parts are connected with each other.

One easiest way is to smile as hard as you can and hold that position for few seconds. Do this effort in three sets of exercise.

Side jaw crunches are another exercise for neck fat loss. Lay your head at one side and pull it as far as you can, the target if to pull the muscles at each side as far as you can do and hold that at each side, repeat it in three sets.

Similar to side jaw crunch, jaw crunches is also the exercise to stretch the neck and trim it within regular workout daily, it works same as abdominal crunches, both of your jaw and neck muscles will stretch. In this, you need to tilt your head backward as far as you can when the neck feels pressure then hold the position for few seconds and then repeat in three-five sets or more as you can do easily.

To firm your neck skin, tilt your head all the sides as far as possible, sideways and then front and back to stretch and hold for couple of seconds each side and continue doing it for few times a day. Try it slowly and maintain for long time.

Try this exercise with your lips and teeth closed, sit or stand in an upright position. Look straight forward and smile as broad as possible. Wait for five seconds and then make your lips pointed in shape without opening them. Hold this kissing position for few seconds and repeat this process 10 times.

Lie straight on your bed and take head to the edge level. Perform this gently by raising your body from head and shoulders till the stomach. After holding this posture for about ten seconds, go back to original position and try five times minimum.

This is an exercise of biggest jaw muscle platysma which joins the jaw to shoulder. It firms chin and throat, all you need to do is with erect spine while sitting or standing pull your lips under teeth and turn corners of mouth down. The neck tendons must stand out and repeat this 5-10 times.

Overall body fat burning

Try mixed cardio grills countless as they are effective enough for you thrice a week. These experiences use variety of muscles in a group of an exercise; they do not wear your body out. Daily use of these drills must be done with care, change intensity of the exercises and reduce the risks of injuries and restlessness. Keep your body in good and balanced condition, first day start with a walk of low intensity and then next day do an intense aerobics activity. Join any class for your ease or take help from visual aids like videos.

Squat is also a fat burning exercise, hold your head straight forward and place feet at the width of shoulders. Bend hips and knees in sitting position; reach lower as you can do easily. Make your arms forward and stretch. Balance yourself while inhale when going down and up when exhale. Then relax your arms at the sides and stand up straight as you were in the beginning.

Do pushups in which you can lie down on floor and open your hand down at the width of the shoulders and on palms, straight your arms gradually and keep your legs and back straight. Inhale while going down to the floor back again and exhale when you move up. Extend your stamina to do them in 2 sets from 15-20 times. This is a hard position but once you start doing it correctly, you will find a great and fast change in your weight.

Raise your legs while lying on the floor straight on back or on stomach, in both the forms, try to move your legs up as much as you can and hold for few seconds. This will stretch both of your legs and tummy, exhale when putting legs to up and inhale when putting down. Return to beginning position after every time you complete a process and repeat 20-30 times a day for best results. Do not do it intensely and slowly when you feel muscle fatigue, relax for some time to stay fine with your muscles.

Arms

Tone your arms to look leaner, try V raise sculpting workout for arms. Hold dumbbells in your each hand and stand with feet at shoulder width. Palms must be at your sides in a position and then stretch arms to forward without locking and raise arms diagonally in front of you. Your arms will then make a V shape and until they are parallel to the floor. Wait for a second and return to original position as you create at the start. Repeat it 12-15 times daily.

Just above your shoulders, hold a pair of dumbbells with standing on feet width apart and bend knees, palms must face each other at that time. Press the dumbbells against each other straight overhead. Hold weights for few seconds and gradually bring dumbbells back to shoulders again and repeat 8-10 times at once. Lower the weight after at least three times of wait above.

Say goodbye to your arm fat for your good, rotating triceps kickback. Bend your knees and stand slightly lean downward. Hold a dumbbell in each hand; bend your right elbow to catch the dumbbell at your side while keeping the upper arm parallel to the floor. Press back the dumbbell and make arms straight, rotate with the palms facing the ceiling and bring back the palm when facing in and then bend the arm again. Complete this move with each arm 12-15 times and get a suitable arm shape without any extra fat and perfect shape.

The focus of this aero cross exercise is shoulders, simply hold ends of ropes in each hand and face palms down, jump through the rope as moving it around your height. This hopping and skipping as you begin will allow you to pass through rope in steps, once you get the rhythm; it passes fast beneath your feet then you can extend your arms width as far as you can and then pass from it. The goal will be to skip big circles and your arms move and stretch clockwise in turn to lose fat and continue it for 60 seconds without break.

Hands & Fingers

Hands and fingers will be slim when you as much as move them in closing and opening ways. Making of fist is the first powerful exercise to remove fats from your palms and fingers. The hands when in motion will get slim and smart. Increase your motions when you are free, make fists again and again and get rid of fats on your hands and fingers which are making your hands ugly, they will also get much range of strength and their stretching makes you feel relieved. Close fists to the tightness whenever you feel free and slowly open them as you will do in any task. You must do it gently or predicts like you are holding something with full grasp. Wrap your thumbs around your fingers fully, this is the simplest stretch to start for your hands and fingers fat. Wait in fist position for almost a minute and then try to release and open your fingers wider. Repeat this fisting exercise about four times in an exercise plan.

Next is fingers stretch and it targets fingers more than hands. Place your hands on a flat table or smooth place straight with palm downward and from that place gently stretch the fingers upward and continue moving up and down back to the surface. Do not force your joints, hold your hand and fingers in upward position for a minute and then moves back to start position, repeat it four times with a hand. Do it with both hands equally.

Another is claw stretch, hold your each hand one by one and try this stretch, keep hand in front of you and make a claw with fingers only and do not move palm, palm must face you while you do this, bend fingertips inward to the direction of palm and touch the base of each finger joint. Your hand will look like a claw then hold for a minute and release back to straight position in front of you and repeat four times with each of your hand.

Hold a small soft ball in your hand and squeeze it on your palm as hard as you can do it easily and then hold for a minute then lose the grip on ball and repeat this with each hand almost 10-15 times, this stretch is not for doing daily, give rest to your hands for 2 days in between. Try it 2-3 times a week.

Similar to above one there is another exercise which is pinch strengthener, take a soft ball of foam and pinch in a hand with each finger one by one with a hold of a minute for each and do it 10-15 times for each hand but same caution is in it to try only twice or thrice a week and give rest to hands of 48 hours, the best is to include these types of hand exercises two days a week with mixing other exercises rest of the week. Change and combine different exercises for different parts and combine to break boredom and enjoy changes with variety and combinations.

Finger lift is another best solution to keep fingers fat away, place your hand flat on a smooth surface and then one by one lift a finger from hand, do it with all the fingers and hold slowly. Complete same with other hand on a table and perform 8-12 times with each hand, you might lift all fingers of a hand together and place palm stick to the surface.

Then there is thumb extension to stretch hands, instead of grabbing, your hand muscles will also feel light when you stretch each of the fingers in hand away from each other, try with stretching of thumbs only away from other fingers, shifts thumbs of each hands one by one opposite to fingers direction, you can do it freely but also you can place hand on a table and wrap a rubber band around the hand to gather fingers together. The base of hand will be down and slowly move thumb away from fingers and hold for 30 or 60 seconds and then set it back, repeat for 15 times and for the health of joints, stay for 48 hours before starting this exercise again.

Back

Kick out the fat at your back with these exercises, repeat this 10 times, take a Swiss ball and lie on it with facedown on the top, make sure your back is flat and your chest is out of the ball surface, hang your arms down the ball straight and keep your shoulders above while make your palms facing each other and arms are hanging down straight. At an angle of 30 degrees, from your bodies raise the arms in Y position. Make arms line with your body and then put them back to the starting point and repeat nine more times.

Repeat this exercise for back 12 times, take a pair of dumbbells and grab them in your hands, bend downward to the floor till hips your torso are parallel to the floor. Let the dumbbells hanged to the floor from your shoulders, your hands face down and palms face each other, do not move your torso and raise your arms in the line of your body to the sides. Take a break at the point and then gradually return from where you start and take break again to complete all repetitions afterwards.

Try modified inverted row, lie on the floor with your face up and secure the shoulders directly under the bar bell. Grab the bar with both hands and move up without moving your feet with knees bend at 90 degrees. Feet will look flat on floor and hips move upward only. Bar bell is at your width and when your chest becomes closer to them, moves back slowly, release and break to relax and repeat five times minimum.

Repeat this last move of negative chin-up five times, set a bench under the bar and step on bench to grab bar with shoulders straight, cross your ankles behind you and wait till your chest is closer to the width of your hands, jump up and down and wait for five seconds before your step again on bench back till your arms are straight again and repeat four more times in a day.

Do each of the above for only twice a week and shift to another for rest of the week for healthy loss and do not forget to take a break between each set of a move of 2 minutes and between each move for 60 seconds and then continue again.

Abdomen

Check out bicycle pose as good way to lose fat from your abdomen. Lie on the floor or set a mat below you, place yourself straight with face up and hands behind your head, support your head lightly with your fingers. Bring your knees to the chest by lifting the blades of your shoulders upward but do not put pressure on your neck. Carefully rotate yourself to the left side and bring the elbow of right side to the knee of opposite side and let the leg straightened. Then continue same pose with the other side, switch and move left elbow to the right leg, keep doing it the pedaling movements with reps of 12-16 and then continue within 1-3 sets.

Captain's chair is the name of this move for abdomen. Hold the handles of a chair while standing on it with face side outward. Make your upper body stable, let the shoulders relax and press back against the pad. Start bending your knees with insertion of pressure on hips to move them up and when they reach to the hip level simply do not arch or pull, swing it up more. Gradually lower back place down feet on the floor and repeat 16 times in sets of 1-3. It is mostly present in gyms but you can do it at home yourself with care and on a stable place.

Ball crunch is another abdomen exercise, you need a ball to do this exercise daily, lie on it with position of your back on the ball and weight on your lower back to cross arms over your chest or place behind your head. Lift your torso over the ball and contract your abs while pulling down your ribcage down to the hips, curl up but make sure that the ball will not move, stay stable and without rolling lower the back down. You will feel the stretch at the abs, repeat it 12-16 times and complete sets of 1-3. The exercises will ball are much more effective than the floor.

In vertical leg crunch, you need to lie on floor and extend your legs upward straight with knees crossed. Keep your hands at the back of head for support but do not pull neck. Lift blades of the shoulders off the floor and contract abs, reach your chest toward the feet. Keep your legs fixed, you will feel a stretch at your belly button as you move up in this move, your spine is up at the top with this movement, repeat it in 1-3 sets with 12-16 times of lower move.

Long arm crunch is one more exercise in abs section, place a mat on floor and lie straight on it with face up, make sure you are on smooth surface and lie straight. Clasp hands behind head with arms near the ears. Do not stress the neck but if you feel the stress you can extend one hand and lower to repeat it in the sets of 1-3 for 12-16 reps. You may hold a dumbbell to add intensity in your moves.

Also try reverse crunch for abs, lie on floor and place hands behind head, you can also place hands on floor and then from lie straight, shift yourself at 90 degrees by bending knees and moving chest up with feet closer together and crossed, curl yourself up and make hips off the floor, take very small movements and swing legs to create momentum. Repeat 15 times in 2 sets.

Lastly, here is crunch with a heel push, lie on the back, bend knees and cradle head with hands. Keep flexing your feet and contract the abs, keep doing it and lift your shoulders off the floor. Do not pull neck with hands and keep hands behind head to support only, when at the top of crunch just press the heels at the floor and against mat to raise the glutes off. Lower and do 15 reps in two sets.

Facts:

The weight is not something you can control but only the food intake can be controlled by you.

You cannot fight diseases without doing friendship with your food.

Stay happy with what you eat or stay happy with what you gain, choice is yours!

A recent study tells about weight loss with vegan diet containing high carbohydrates and low fats with moderate protein. This diet targets women more than men but both genders get benefits in one way or the other. This diet for weight loss also improves insulin sensitivity, your lifestyle will be active than before and walk for long miles will not be an issue, the respiration improves and health too. This new study was revealed by a September issue in 2013 by *The American Journal of Medicine*. A large number of studies have showed the relation between vegan diet and weight loss, obesity and weight gain is rarely seen in those who follow vegan diet. In a Swedish study by Tufts University researcher P. Kirstin Newby and her colleagues, results showed that those who are meat eaters were obese and the vegan eaters were smart. The study was done on about 55000 people. Throughout the world, the vegans are less at risk of diabetes, heart disease and other health issues. The life of vegans is free of life threatening experiences. Vegan diet is free of all those things that triggers weight gain and invites diseases. This diet does not allow someone to stay hungry and restless. More dietary fiber is present in this diet. They are healthy in losing weight. Cut down on fats and concentrate on getting fit by focusing on getting rid of fried foods and spreads, all of the fast foods, commercial and outside foods are full of fats and do not contain freshness. Try to consume plenty of veggies and fruits. Finally increase the activity level and adopt a habit of doing walk for one hour, cycling, sports and other activities. This is not a formula for instant weight loss but slowly and steadily everything will be better and in shape. Your muscles will build up with energy and not fats, the proportion of your body parts will set and try to start your day with fiber breakfasts. Replace every bad food with healthy food and consume only the foods which are welcome in vegan diet, chew on plants and mix in the leaves under your smoothies and shakes. This diet is a lot better than meat based and any other diets in the matter of weight loss. Positive benefits will be seen after you try it and stick to it for couple of months, the visible difference then asks you to continue for years.

Use of organic foods are healthy for you, they are real foods to use when you are conscious about your health and weight, include organic foods in your diet for better weight loss plan results. Organic foods are quite healthier and strong for people on diet plan as compared to conventional foods and it can easily be viewed through an increase in the growth of organic food industry in recent 6 years. The 30% of increase tells us that how people in environmental groups are now supporting and accepting organic foods. No one wants damage of pesticides and fertilizers in their body and safe food is the desire of all consumers, to accomplish it organic foods are best. Everyone is promoting organic foods in the markets; experts are in the view that the uses of these foods are good for weight loss as compared to low fat and soy products. These foods are free of any use of chemicals in their production and growth. Their producers are highly strong contributors in the promotion of organic foods among population; anyone who is a supporter of healthy and natural environment supports organic foods. There are a lot of accurate data to explain that how these foods are good for your health. In the previous years, the products were misrepresented and from recent years few scientific evidences showed their quality and effectiveness on human body and healthy lifestyle. Small amounts of proofs are present about few organic products but still the varieties of foods in organic category are better than others especially the milk and tomatoes. FDA and USDA did not mention them better than non-organic foods but actually they are better according to researches done on them.

What is better in organic milk? The researchers showed that organic milk contains large amounts of antioxidants, CLA, vitamins and Omega 3 fatty acids than present in regular foods. Cows who give organic milk are pasture grazed and this is the reason that organic milk is better than non-organic milk (The Danish Institute of Agricultural Research at the University of Aberdeen and the Institute of Grassland and Environmental Research) the organic milk has better quality.

In the matter of organic tomatoes, the University of California conducted a study, in which Davis the researcher concluded after ten years of study that the tomatoes which are organic have grown in environment which is rich in nutrients and low in nitrogen rich chemicals and this leads to 79% higher amounts of antioxidants and excessive formation of quercetin and kaempferol. Antioxidants are essential for us in the prevention of cardiovascular diseases, cancers and overall reduction in health issues. According to the studies on organic foods, mankind should stop growing foods other than organic environment but it is not possible for everyone because they are usually high price procedures and not every farmer can afford which in turn cause increase in prices of the products in developing countries and developing countries cannot buy them much. Any study did not prove that without the use of chemicals and fertilizers the toxic bacteria and harmful viruses invade food substances but it is not true. No one can deny the benefits of organic foods, there are plenty of useful claims due to organic farming practices. They are:

Reduction in pesticides

Great capacity of antioxidants

Good for immunity and heart

Resistant to antibiotics

Better taste

Best for overall health

Safe for environment

It is assumed that vegan diet accelerates weight loss if the ratio of dairy and meat products is set to minimum. The diet plan with the use of vegan foods five days a week and other foods only on weekends are good for health and weight loss. Fatty foods when used less and in controlled amounts cause you to stay fit and leaner than others and than those who use these fatty foods regularly. The rate of weight loss in vegans is determined as two pounds loss per week which is not a bad deal. Use nuts when you need crunch in your mouth instead of heave desserts and commercial cookies and snacks simply eat one oz. of walnuts and stay fit.

Quotes

They are best for inspiration:

"If food is your best friend, it's also your worst enemy."
~Edward "Grandpa" Jones

"Processed foods not only extend the shelf life, but they extend the waistline as well." ~Karen Sessions

"Don't dig your grave with your own knife and fork."
~English Proverb

"No matter who you are, no matter what you do, you absolutely, positively do have the power to change." ~Bill Phillips

"Probably nothing in the world arouses more false hopes than the first four hours of a diet." ~Dan Bennett

"Believe and act as if it were impossible to fail." ~Charles F. Kettering

"If you don't like something, change it. If you can't change it, change your attitude. Don't complain." ~Maya Angelou

"Animals are my friends...and I don't eat my friends."
— George Bernard Shaw

"A man can live and be healthy without killing animals for food; therefore, if he eats meat, he participates in taking animal life merely for the sake of his appetite. And to act so is immoral."
— Leo Tolstoy

"It is my view that the vegetarian manner of living, by its purely physical effect on the human temperament, would most beneficially influence the lot of mankind."
— Albert Einstein

"You're thinking I'm one of those wise-ass California vegetarians who is going to tell you that eating a few strips of bacon is bad for your health. I'm not. I say it's a free country and you should be able to kill yourself at any rate you choose, as long as your cold dead body is not blocking my driveway."
— Scott Adams

"I have from an early age abjured the use of meat, and the time will come when men such as I will look upon the murder of animals as they now look upon the murder of men."
— Leonardo da Vinci

"People often say that humans have always eaten animals, as if this is a justification for continuing the practice. According to this logic, we should not try to prevent people from murdering other people, since this has also been done since the earliest of times."
— Isaac Bashevis Singer

"I can't count the times that upon telling someone I am vegetarian, he or she responded by pointing out an inconsistency in my lifestyle or trying to find a flaw in an argument I never made. (I have often felt that my vegetarianism matters more to such people than it does to me.)"
— Jonathan Safran Foer, *Eating Animals*

Tricks

Eat only when you are hungry.

Eat food of the size of your palm or a fist.

Do not eat starters at a restaurant or completely eliminate dining out.

Do not eat in a standing position.

Eat foods at room temperature to cold temperatures.

Check labels of foods each time you shop.

Replace artificial snacks with natural raw foods.

Take only a spoon of dessert/sweet on special occasions.

Fill your meals with veggies as possible.

Never eat dessert, soda drinks and other white sugar foods empty stomach.

Use meal replacement smoothies instead of meals often.

Set a goal to achieve healthy lifestyle including physical activity and eating as a target with the change in underlying causes of related thoughts and beliefs.

Seek experienced advises along with professional, not only doctors and counselors but someone who had history of binge eating control and successful treatments are good ones too.

Maria Simonson, ScD, PhD, director of the Health, Weight, and Stress Clinic at the Johns Hopkins Medical Institutions in Baltimore gave a logical idea to binge on spicy foods, sauces and spices than savor, bland and sweet foods because they satisfy your faster in turn helps you stop eating and also burn your calories at a faster rate. Chili peppers and Tabasco sauce are just the examples to add in foods also lemon juice and pickles works good.

After limiting your portion size, keep it in mind that anything cannot be happen within days by moving a magic wand.

Include yoga, machines stuff, sports, playing tennis, boxing, basketball, running, dumbbells, use of ropes, jumps, walking, running, climbing stairs and anything you can do alone.

Always keep your self-esteem higher and do not think badly about yourself just because of your shape. Always remember the happy times, achievements, praises, good qualities, positivity and successes. You can do it by doing your weigh frequently without much effort, throw the scale out.

Dress yourself in dark fitted clothes and in which you feel comfortable and good to yourself. Walk confidently around people and think mostly about your good body parts. Groom yourself daily as first thing in the morning and get rid of skinny and light clothes.

Adopt a pet and spend time with it in playing, walking and talking.

Sleep well and completely 8 hours a day in calm environment. Make yourself clean, take warm bath and talk supportive with everyone so you will get back the same to keep yourself motivated.

Watch movies or long TV programs which interests you without grabbing food or at eating time. Listen good music for hours.

Participate in home tasks throughout the day even cooking but do not pick something to your mouth during the whole process.

Avoid yourself from alcohol in all means, occupy yourself after each meal for 4-6 hours and fix your meals to number of times.

Do not leave yourself hungry and never join a party night without eating and with empty stomach.

Volunteer in similar causes, join a music band or activity, join art competition, speech and debating competitions, plan your grouping times, change groups and longtime conversations with relations you have.

Always think that whatever you are doing is right except eating. Be assertive and up to date.

Review your strengths and do not judge your figure, simply complain less and accept more, in a quiet time stay positive. To be angry is also normal; accomplish your wishes with checklists.

Once you are done with eating, stop thinking that you will gain weight and move more.

Set realistic goals for your daily eating and feel the sense of accomplishment when achieved. Reward yourself after every loss.

Stay active but do not look more at fashion magazines because they makes you away from reality and enables you to fantasize more about your ideal figure but struggle less on the goals.

Use fat burning foods:

Whey

Beans and legumes

Whole grains

Spinach and green veggies

Berries

Chili peppers

Green tea

Nuts

Enova oil

Nut butters

Fatty fish or salmon

Grapefruit

Lemon

Oats

Lentils and veggies

Water

Remedies

Consume an apple daily.

Daily eat a citrus fruit or take a cup of citrus fruit juice empty stomach.

Season foods with chilies and cayenne peppers.

Use dairy products without fat.

Take cabbage or tomato soup daily.

Use cardamom and curry leaves.

Drink herbal green tea daily.

Use meal replacement or green smoothies with fiber.

Adopt physically active life with simple exercises.

Use fish oils in your foods.

There are a number of positive results with the use of these strategies, so Good Luck!